BORROWED ANGEL

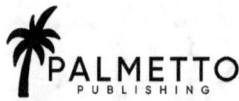

Charleston, SC
www.PalmettoPublishing.com

Borrowed Angel
Copyright © 2022 by Drake Gaetano

All rights reserved

No portion of this book may be reproduced, stored in a retrieval system, or transmitted in any form by any means–electronic, mechanical, photocopy, recording, or other–except for brief quotations in printed reviews, without prior permission of the author.

First Edition

Paperback ISBN: 979-8-8229-0151-3
eBook ISBN: 979-8-8229-0152-0

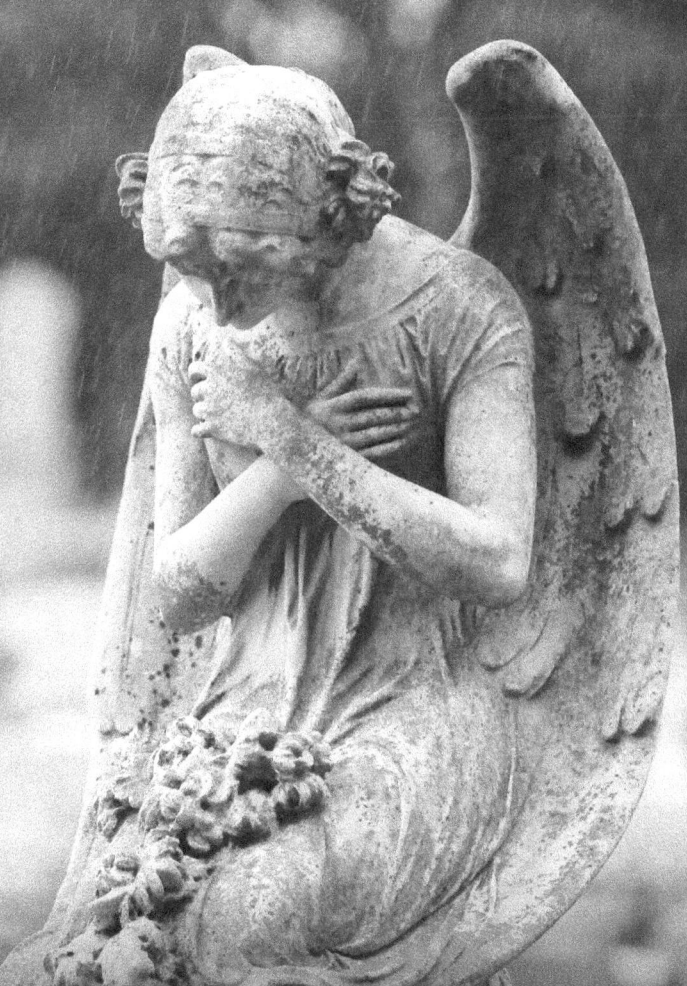

BORROWED ANGEL

DRAKE GAETANO

Dedication

I dedicate this book to the loving memory of Jason Michael Coughlin, and to his mother Elaine Margaret Coughlin, for their bravery at a time when despite a grim prognosis, they held onto a thread of hope until the end.

Acknowledgement

I am deeply moved and eternally grateful to Elaine Margaret Coughlin for allowing me to write her story; one that has helped her through the process of grieving after suffering a most devestating loss.

Table of Contents

Synopsis 1

Borrowed Angel 3

Epilogue 35

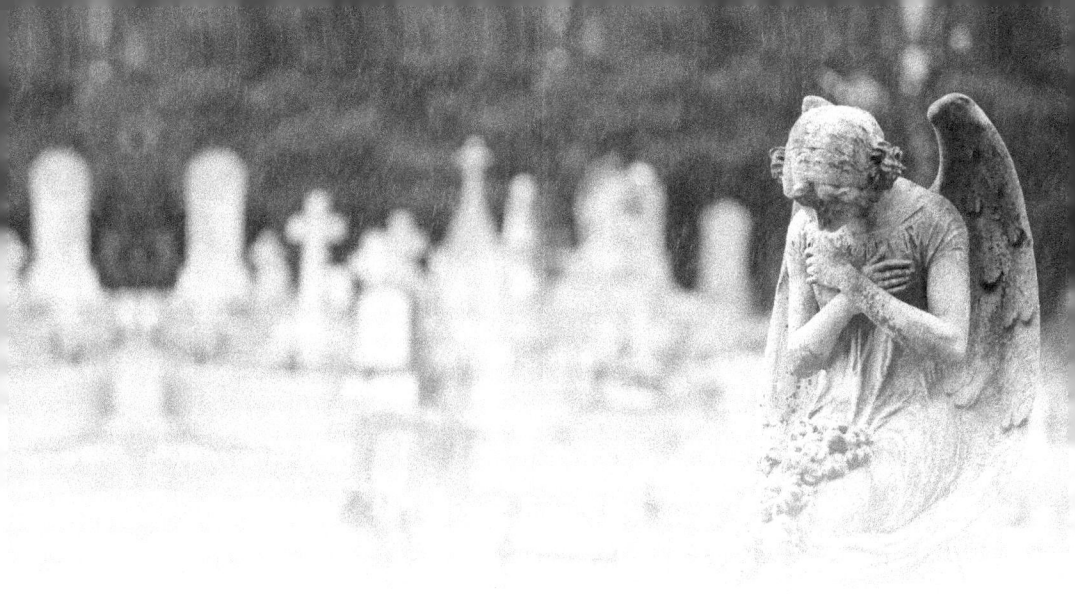

Synopsis

Losing a loved one inevitably results in perpetual, incalculable, grief, and there is no loss greater for a mother than to lose a child — no less an only son. This compelling story concerns a mother who never allows fear and hopelessness to cast a shadow of doubt over her belief in miracles, the power and sanctity of God, and an inevitability of life which is inviolate.

When discovering her son Jason was diagnosed with a rare form of lung cancer, Elaine prepared herself for the remaining precious time they would have together. But those years were filled with anxiety and trepidation while she watched his life slowly begin to ebb away. After her three month stay in the hospital, she discovered what she had known all along; that life is precious and can't be redeemed by assumptions, empty words, or promises, and if angels really do exist, they went unnoticed in room 420.

Based on true life events, Borrowed Angel, will open your heart to the the pain, suffering, and healing of a mother who lost the one thing in life that she loved most. It may help the reader to see that angels are real, then, that they can mend a broken heart, and despite what others may believe, are servants of a higher being.

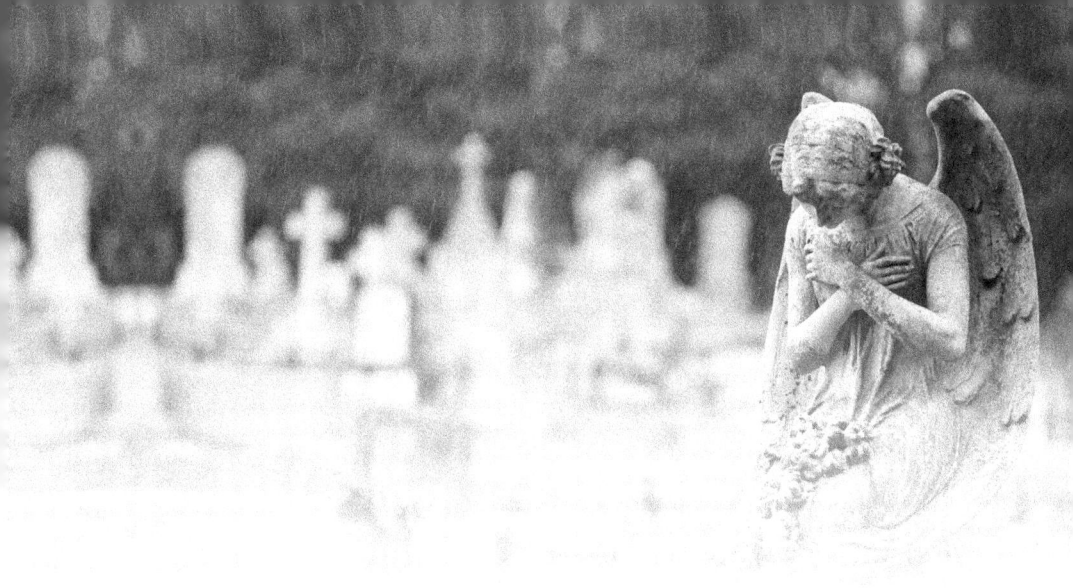

Borrowed Angel

The ambulance ride was agonizing. Elaine held her son's hand while she prayed over him, watching him struggle to catch what she hoped wouldn't be his last breath. She thought; *Was he loosing his final battle for his life? He can't be, I won't let him! Can't this ambulance go any faster? Why is it taking so damn long to get to the hospital? This is an emergency, can't they see that! He's my baby, he can't die. God, please don't let him die, he's too young.*

"Try not to worry ma'am, the hospital's just around the corner." Assuring words for a much needed moment of repose.

Finally, she though, as she gazed at the hospital staff awaiting Jason's arrival. They moved him quickly down the corridor toward the emergency room to begin life support. She followed close by, frightened and alone. The scene inside the ER was "hands on", while the doctor and nurses worked to get oxygen into his starving lungs. The attending doctor looked at Elaine and said, "If you want your son to survive, you must leave this room. "Now!" (Jason was dying from stage three Adenocarcinoma lung cancer).

Her mind raced with fear and anxiety while she paced the corridor, praying and hoping that each step would bring some relief. It didn't. *He's only 39 years old. He's all I've got. Please, God, don't let him die.* But was God listening to her pleas? Would he spare her beloved son?

She sat in the waiting room while wild thoughts of despair distracted her from her prayers. She walked the corridor and prayed, and prayed some more. Thoughts of pending doom kept filling her head. She fought harder to resist. Sitting with a profound feeling of nausea, she continued to ask God for strength. It was 11:00 p.m. and sadness, fear, and total desperation were at their peak.

Frantic notions raced inside of her head, leaving her to feel like she was drowning in an ocean of anxiety, and despair. *My God, when will I find something out? She needed to stay hopeful and strong. Jason mustn't see her any other way. For him, for him, I need to do it for him, I must stay strong. Whatever I do, I can't cry in front of him. I must stay strong, for his sake. She repeated those words over and over. God, give me strength. You promised never to give me more than I could bear. How long will I have to wait? This is killing me!"*

She sat, walked, and waited some more. At 4 a.m., she heard footsteps. It was the doctor. She met her in the hallway. She was the same pulmonologist that had seen Jason the day before.

She said, "Jason is on life support, but his body's shutting down. His airways are closing off and he's not getting enough oxygen to survive. There's not much we can do for him here anymore.

"You have two choices. Once we get him stabilized, you can move him to a hospice facility, or we can try to keep him alive here for as long as we can. Either way, there are no guarantees that he will survive."

"How long could that be doctor?"

"Maybe a few hours, weeks, maybe longer. There's no telling, it depends on his will to live."

They walked the hallway to room 420. Elaine thought; *No, we are not giving up. I know Jason wouldn't want it any other way. We will walk these steps together no matter what. There's no reason for things to change now.* Once inside, the urge to cry fostered its undenying intent within seconds. *I can do this. I need to do this. I need to stay strong, Jason musn't see me cry.* The only way Jason could communicate was with his eyes, mouthing his words, and hand gestures.

She glanced out the window into a vanishing rainbow, and a sky that opened up to a bright sun and panoramic view of a large body of water, rolling hills, and a small small flower garden. It gave her the time she needed to gather her composure before facing Jason. She followed the path of a small flock of sparrows until one of them withdrew from the group and landed on the branch of a tree sitting in the middle of the garden. It sat there for a second, hopped onto a stone statue, before resting on a nearby bench. Her eyes withdrew when she caught site of Jason lying with a plastic ventilation tube to prevent possible asphyxiation.

The doctor spoke, "We can administer five more treatments of radiation, but there's no guarantee they will help."

Elaine looked at Jason and said, "I think it's worth a try Jason". Is that what you want to do?"

He nodded yes. The doctor admitted him and immediately began the round of treatments. She looked back at Jason. He was crying. She knew that it was not for himself, but for her.

Food and liquids were administered through an IV tube, while their only way to communicate was through eye contact, an occasional written note, and the small success they had reading each other's lips. Elains faith in God, and her hope for a complete recovery never dwindled. God's presence was the only solace that was felt between them. She would never know what was really going on inside of Jason's head. *Was he having conversations with God, or was he only living in an agonizing wasteland of terror and doubt? Only he and God would know that. She only wanted things to get better, or just get it over with.*

During that first night, Elaine's memory drifted back to the time of Jason's diagnosis. When she heard the prognosis, she decided that with the time they had left, they would take a trip. She wanted him to visit the wayside chapels in small villages, the surrounding countryside, and the remains of an ancient chapel on the castle grounds of St John The Baptist church on the island of Alicudi off the coast of Sicily. They became "prayer warriors", asking God to heal Jason and to give them the peace, strength, and hope to see things through together. They had been inseparable since he was a baby, why should things be any different now? It was always just her and Jason. That's the way it always was, and that's the way it would remain. Besides, God was always with her and Jason, and knew what was best for both of them — to live a long life together; one that would last for all eternity. With Jason's health rapidly deteriorating, she wrapped herself in a cloak of hope, while God hands shielded Jason's body. No longer could a mothers love protect her son from what seemed a certain death. Jason remained intubated for the next seventeen days with only a single tube connected to his windpipe that was keeping him alive. She sat alone in room 420, in a state of severe and prolonged anxiety, anticipating each breath that Jason struggled to take. She watched the sun peek its head slightly above the horizon, while once again, a group of sparrows flew into view. As if by command, a sparrow left the flock, landed on the same branch, the same stone statue, before coming to rest on the same bench as before.

The doctor entered, interrupting Elaine's inkling that perhaps this was a message that she needed to pay attention to.

With a cold voice, she said, "We would like to try five radiation treatments, but in my opinion, it won't help" — words that left a sting on any ray of hope that Jason would survive for much longer. It wasn't a death sentence, but it was quite frightening.

In the weeks to come, Elaine came to know the hospital as a place of healing. Soothing colors, natural light, pleasant sounds, and the surrounding visual stimuli helped to somewhat reduce her anxiety. Exposure to views of nature, interior and exterior gardens, aquariums, and art with a nature theme brought her solace and hope. A meditation room provided a refuge provided a meditation room to pray.

She cried out, "The air that I breathe is your holy presence living in me, my Lord Jesus. I am desperate for you, and every word that you speak to me. I'm lost without you. "I pray that you hear my voice dear Lord."

There were other tiny places of peace and reflection that she visited when she felt her heart could no longer bear the pain. Once a week, her sisters came, knowing that it might be that it might be their last time they would see their nephew. One day, he handed a note to one of his aunts; *Please take care of my mother after I'm gone, she's going to need you. I love you.*

Sunday mornings always began with a visit from a priest. Then, like clockwork, Elaine's best friend Terri came to visit, hoping to boost her spirits and relieve her for a while so she could take care of things needing her attention. On several occasions, Elaine spent time reflecting in the garden outside of room 420. She was intrigued by the arrival of a sparrow every time she entered the garden. She wondered if it just a coincidence that it arrived at the exact time she did, only to take flight the second she got up to leave? As a Christian, she believed that Jesus spoke of the sparrow in a way that would seem strange and even delusional to some. He chose the sparrow as a simple illustration of his abiding love.

Behold the fowls of the air; for they sow not neither, do they reap, nor gather into barns; yet your heavenly father feedeth them. I will instruct thee and teach thee in the way which thou shall go; I will guide thee with mine eye.

Suddenly the thought that Jason might die while she was gone, prompted her to head back up to his room. With her mind racing, she kept repeating the words; "Keep your eye on the sparrow, keep your eye on the sparrow", keep your eye on the sparrow." She became less anxious, and thanked God for his intervention.

With the entrance hall just up ahead, the soothing notes of a piano interrupted her silent lamentation. They reached parts of her soul that were previously unexplored but now willingly accepted. Each note reached out and spoke to her, drawing her closer to a beautiful young girl, about nineteen years old, seated in the middle of the room at a grand piano. She sat with the poise and grace of a concert pianist, captivating Elaine's sense of serenity until the last note was played.

"Such beautiful music played by someone so young." I was on my way back up to my son's room and your music caught my attention and drew me to you."

"Why thank you, I'm glad you liked it. "I wrote it about two years ago", the girl replied. "It was my first song. The lyrics are from my first poem."

"Today was the first day I was brave enough to play it in public. I have written many arrangements since then, but this is still my favorite. I still play it from the original sheet of paper

I wrote it on. I believe God gave me the mind to write the words, and the hands to play the music. It was his gift."

"My name is Linda,

"What's your's?"

"Elaine".

What brings you here Linda?"

"I'm waiting for the results of a barrage of tests. I have breast cancer and it doesn't look good for me."

"My son Jason is in critical condition from lung cancer, and I'm afraid he will soon die."

"I'm so sorry".

Elaine broke the silence, "Jason received some solid piano training when he was young, but he decided not to follow a career in music.
"He received a degree in Art History and English Literature, but he chose to play his high level of music just for the love of it. With Jason, it was never about the money."

Linda asked, "How old is Jason?"

"He just turned 39 in September."

"It was wonderful to meet you, Elaine. I will certainly pray for him."

"Thank you so much Linda. It was wonderful meeting you as well. I hope everything works out well for you. I'll put you in my daily prayers."

"Thank you."

Linda closed the keyboard,"I hope that someday I'll be able to meet Jason."
I only hope I live long enough." Good bye, Elaine."
"Good bye Linda". "Oh, I almost forgot to ask, what inspired you to write that song?"

Linda smiled, "An angel."
She handed Elaine the had written piece of paper, "I've had this long enough, now it belongs to you."

She watched her disappear into the elevator

She sat on a bench nearby and read these words;

Borrowed Angel

You touched our lives in a special way,
—- But all too soon you were called away.
—- And tho' we weep that you could not stay,
—- Your life won't be in vain, we pray.

Borrowed Angel, you've helped us see
—- How precious and fleeting life can be
—- And so our pledge sweet angel to thee
—- Is to treasure life and family

So whisper to our spirits, every now and then
—- Remind us to be worthy time and time again.
—- We promise that we'll hold you, tho" we cannot promise when;
—- Sweet dreams, borrowed angel, until we meet again.

At the bottom it read; *Angels are children on loan from God —* Linda Myers 2008

Elaine said a prayer for Linda, in hopes that the next time she would see her she would be Cancer--free. What a joyful moment that would be. She stopped at the gift shop on her way, and bought an angel of love remembrance for Jason. When she held it up to him, he wept.

There weren't any good days, only those occasionall filled with hope of spending another day watching Jason suffer. God gave Elaine access to an seemingly limitless amount of strength and endurance, knowing that we go through moments in our lives when we must be brave, even when it seems impossible.

She spent her days filled with never-ending struggle. She watched Jason's labored breathing, never stopping to pray or give up hope. Nighttime cast a heavy cloak of hopelessness and doubt upon her, along with her trust in God and all the things she was brought up to believe in. It also allowed for an opportunity to overcome the dread and doubtfulness that plagued her, knowing deep down that she needed to stay strong, patient, and hopeful to allow God the time to do his work. She held on to the angel that she had given to Jason and prayed for Gods intervention.

Many nights, she would get up from twilight sleep and go to Jason's bedside.

She'd hold his hand and say, "I love you so much."

"I know how much you have always loved me, and I know that our love will go on forever, even after you leave me."

"I know that someday both of us will be in the arms of God, and I will always hold on to you in the depths of my heart, and I'll never, ever, let you go."

He couldn't talk, but his eyes spoke with an assurance that he understood everything she was saying, and that everything was going to be okay.

It was 2 a.m. when she went and sat in the garden, hoping to ease her mind. Several of the night staff were coming and going, and she wondered if any of them might be on their way to Jason's room. She thought; *people come and go here, but there was nothing more they could do to change Jason's date with death.* God was in charge of that. She tried desperately to rid her mind of thoughts of impending doom. Her intention to go there was to soothe her mind, not to deepen her sorrow. She went back upstairs.

Inside, she saw a young woman waiting for an elevator.

Once inside, the girl asked, "What floor would you like?"

"Four please."

"That's the same floor I'm getting off on. "My mother's in room 426."

"She's just a few rooms down the hall from my son. "How long has your mother been in the hospital?"

"I've been searching just about every hospital in the country for her. I finally tracked her down here yesterday."

She's being treated for severe drug addiction."

"What's going on with you?"

"My son is very ill with lung cancer, he's not expected to live."

"Oh, I'm so sorry, I shouldn't have asked. Please forgive me."

"That's ok."

"How's your mother doing?"

"She's battling everyday to stay alive, but she's hanging in there. "She's been plagued by drug addiction and diabetes her whole life, and honestly I'm sick and tired of her shenanigans."

"She's getting just what she deserves.

"She's already lost one of her legs, and God only knows what's next." My brothers a pilot. He flies his own plane. He's waiting for me at the airport to find out if I found her here. I hope he doesn't leave without me like he did once before."

"I don't know what to do."

"Maybe praying will do the trick." I've never been one for prayer, but maybe it's about time to find out if it really works."

If she dies, I"ll know it doesn't."

Elaine asked, "Can I walk you to your mothers room so we can talk a little more"? I would like to tell you something."

"Sure."

"This is Jason's room."

He's my only child, and was in his twenties when he his drug addiction began."

Please try not to blame your mother, try to forgive her."

"It wasn't something she planned on."

"She just lost control of her life like Jason did." It can happen to anyone."

"My intentions aren't meant to offend you, and I hope you don't take it the wrong way."

"It's just that I'm a mother, and sometimes children don't know the circumstances that brought their parents to the point of addiction.

"I wish you all the luck in the world. I will pray for you and your mother."

The girl replied, "And I'll pray for Jason."

A few more nights later, two nurses' aides approached Elaine. They heard about the angel, and asked if the could borrow it to pray for a woman in critical condition just down the hall. They returned a short while later, thanked Elaine, and after a brief conversation, left. The next day, two different aids asked for the same near- perfect scenario.

The very next night, the nurse handed her a folded piece of paper. She said, "You just missed a young woman who handed me this and left the room without saying a word."

Elaine said, "That's odd". It read; *Some people come into our lives and quickly disappear. Others stay for a while, make footprints on our heart, leave, and we are never the same.* Signed; an angel.

She said, "Do you remember what she looked like?"

"Was she a patient in the hospital?"

The nurse replied, "She came and went so fast that I didn't get a chance to get a real good look at her."
"But she certainly was beautiful."

"She had the face of an angel."

Elaine was almost certain that it had to have been Linda, the girl she met playin the piano. She felt like she and Jason were being surrounded by guardian angels — and Linda was one of them.

Then Elaine's world came crashing down. Jason got progressively worse, and despite being on the ventilator, the doctor began the process of sedation. His suffering was excruciating. He had fluid in his lungs, blood transfusions, infection, and pulmonary embolus, for which he took antibiotics. His extremities swelled to twice their size, his heart rate would spike to 200+ then plummet, and his blood pressure would soar. Witnessing this was the most traumatic event she could ever have imagined.She became numb when she realized she was losing him.

It was now the morning of September 28, 2010. Jason was successfully sedated, slowly dying as his body began to shut down. The doctor stopped in every few hours to check in on him.

He said, "I think you need to know this." "At some point, Jason's heart will stop beating,
his lungs will burst, and he'll be gone."

Sickening words from an uncaring doctor that no mother should ever be allowed to hear. Things were moving much too quickly, and she wasn't ready to let go of Jason or the dwindling options of chemo.

All she cared about was that Jason was still alive, and she could still hold his hand, kiss his face, and pray with him. She realized now more than ever that his life would come to a sudden end, and all she wanted was to give him everything she had left to give for as long as she could. She poured out her heart and emptied everything she had for him. Jason looked at her and mouthed, "I don't want to die." She lookedat Jason, and with her heart wretched with sadness she said,

"Jason, there's nothing more the doctors can do for you, you're are going to die." Suddenly, she realized that only through the grace of God, Jason was delivered into this world, and that she was now prepared for him to be taken from her, and placed into the loving hands of God. As long as his years of suffering would end and he would be with the Lord for all eternity, then his death would be a blessing.

She knew that the rays of light shining upon him from heaven, would now separate him from his earthly mother, and with no regrets knew that the things that he touches in Heaven will be far greater than the things he left behind.

She whispered, "Goodbye my darling son. "Your real treasure lies just beyond the end of a rainbow." Now only the respirator would keep him alive. He refused to have it shut down. He was petrified of suffocation and in his decision he wrote' "I will die from Cancer, not suicide."

There was nothing else to do but to try and comfort her dearly beloved son. She felt the same torment as the blessed Mother watching her son die in excruciating pain and suffering. She just wanted the suffering to stop.

In those last two days, Jason struggled to breathe, desperately trying to cry out to his mother. He could no longer stand the pain. In those last hours, he was heavily sedated while his mother continued to play music and sing songs as she wiped his swollen and sweaty body with ice. She was taking care of her baby boy once again, only this time she was preparing him to die. From the very beginning, she realized her life would only be fulfilled by Jason.

Around 6am, a severe thunderstorm erupted right outside his room. It's presence seemed like a preordained display of God's mighty power. Once it had moved on, the sky was filled with a beautiful rainbow that seemed to reach far toward heaven. The critical care nurse entered the room and turned the bed toward the window while Jason lapsed in and out of consciousness.

The nurse placed her hands on Elaines shoulders and said,

"Did you see the monitor?"

"No."

Jasons body lay motionless.

She knew he was gone. The respirator was no longer keeping him alive. She laid herself across his body, caressing the son she had committed her life to. He was now at the threshold of his new eternal home. His faith in God had released him from death's final grip — his destiny had been fulfilled.

Elaine sat silently crying and praying to God, but Jason's time on earth had run out. He died on September 28, 2010, two years after he was diagnosed with such a dreaded disease.

The nurses allowed her all the time she needed. When they did come in, she stayed to make sure they would be gentle with Jason's body. She remained in constant prayer, trying to hold herself together until the funeral director arrived. With a shattered soul, she touched and kissed Jason, never taking her hands off of her dearly beloved son.

After they took him away she collected his belongings and removed the many get well cards from the walls. She remembered how she read them every day. The one thing she couldn't find was the angel piece that she gave to him. She remembered placing it on the table next to Jason so that an angel would always be close by. She tried to think of reasons why it was missing, but for whatever reason it was gone.

She read the words he wrote on a piece of paper the day before; when I'm gone, I want you to go on with your life and be happy. Don't do anything stupid.

Even though broken-hearted, the last few words brought a smile to her face. That was Jason. She put the paper back in her purse and left.

A few weeks later she returned to the hospital as a way to begin closure, and at the same time to see if anyone might have found the angel piece that came up missing. She hadn't thought about it much since Jason passed, but she did believe it was worth checking into. A wave of mixed emotions swept over her when she came upon the garden where she had spent so much time. Might she get a glimpse of a sparrow? She hoped so. An elderly woman sat on the bench appearing to be in an agitated state of distress.

"Please don't feel like I'm intruding, but are you alright? Do you need some help?" Elaine asked.

The woman looked up and said,

"Thank you for your concern my dear, but I'll be Ok."

"Are you sure? I'd be more than happy to help".

"There's not much anyone can do for me now."

She pointed toward thel window and said,

"My granddaughters up there, and she's gravely ill."

"I came down here to get away for a little while and pray that she survives the day".

"I'm so sorry, I will pray for her. What room is she in?" Asked Elaine.

"Room 420, The woman replied."

"She's so young and has such a talent for writing music and poetry. Her first love has always been the piano."

"By any chance might her name be Linda?" asked Elaine.

"Why yes, do you know her?"

"Yes, at least I think I do.

"I stopped one day awhile ago to listen to a young girl who was playing the piano in the entrance hall. She told me her name was Linda." "We only spent a brief time together, but she left a lasting impression on me."

"She said that she was here because she was dealing with Cancer, and I got the impression that she wasn't very hopeful."

"We talked a little more, and as she was leaving, she gave me a paper with the words to a song she had written a long time ago."

"She said that the words were from a poem she had also written.

Sobbing, the woman said,

"That's Linda, that's my granddaughter. She's such a caring soul. An angel from god is what most everyone said about her".

"And she's just that, an angel. I don't want to see her die. She's too young, and she has so much more life to live and so much more love to give."

"She's always been my little angel."

'I'm on my way up there now to take care of a few things," replied Elaine.

"I hope and pray that everything turns out well for her; and for you as well. God bless you both."

Elaine headed up to room 420.

She stopped at the nurses station to inquire about the gift that disappeared from Jason's room. The nurse looked through a bunch of things before saying, "

"Is this what you're looking for?"

"Yes. Thank you so much, I'm so glad someone found it." .

Elaine passed room 420 envisioning the last thing that Jason saw before he died — a beautiful rainbow. She believed that somewhere beyond the grave there is a land where Jesus went to prepare a resting place. Some people called it Heaven. It was now the place that Jason would call home. In her heart she knew that when heaven came into view, Jason would see that the best was yet to come.

She stopped back at the nurses station to enquire if she could visit Linda. The nurse checked and said (she) would be unable to have a visitor at that time. She asked for a pencil and paper and wrote; Dear Linda, I will be praying for you while God watches over you. Thank you for borrowed angel. Signed, an angel. She headed back to the garden hoping that Linda's grandmother was still there. She was.

The woman said,

"I can't begin to tell you how much comfort you brought me when you stopped by just now."

Elaine told her that she tried to see her, but was told it wasn't a good time.

She handed her the angel and said,

"She's a borrowed angel, and now she belongs to Linda." Life is too short and we're all here on borrowed time."

The woman replied, "Oh how wonderful. You are so kind. I'll go right up now and give it to her. "Lifes real treasures do lie just beyond the rainbow."

"God bless you my dear." You yourself, are certainly one of God's angels". May God always bless you always."

Jason was laid to rest in Syracuse New York, where he'd lived his entire life. His mother, Elaine, moved to Florida as soon as arrangements were made for someone to look after his gravesite. When Jason died, a part of her died, also, leaving only pieces of a shattered life Even in her grief, she saw him smiling, laughing, and at times, she smelled the scent of his soul. She often thought back to the first time she held her baby, looked deep into his eyes … and discovered God. She remains a person of faith, honor, and perpetual illumination to those fortunate enough to cross her path.

She visited his gravesite once more before leaving, placing a single red rose on his headstone. She caught the reflection of something on the ground, and picked up the angel half buried among the blades of grass — an angel that she believed was lost forever. She wondered how such a thing was possible? She thought back to the grandmother she had met at the Hospitol on her way out, but how could it have made its way back to his gravesite? Somehow, they woman must have found out. Nothing else made any sence, but it was cause enough for her. She knelt in prayer.

A woman close by asked, "Are you all right?"
"Yes, thank you, I just found something near and dear to me That I thought was gone forever."
The woman said, "It must have special meaning."

"Yes, it was a gift I gave to my son."

"How touching. I'm so glad to know that you found such a wonderful treasure."

Elaine handed the angel to the woman and said, "I know we just met, and we may never meet again, but I would like for you to accept this. It may help to ease the pain of losing your loved one."
"Angels have a way of easing our pain."

"Oh no, please, I couldn"t accept it, it means too much to you."

Elaine replied,"Perhaps we will meet someday and you can return it. If not, please pass it on to someone else."
"God is good and protects his own, and no one but angels can deliver his messages.
She walked away assured that life's most priceless treasures are delivered on his time.

The end.

Epilogue

The most beautiful people are those who struggle, suffer, and have healed through the realm of agony and uncertainty. Those who have known loss, have found their way out of the depths of despair and have risen above a lifetime of sorrow. Those seasons of sustained doubt and unhappiness, have taught them an abundance of gratitude, sensitivity, and an understanding of life that fills them with compassion, gentleness, and a deep loving concern for others.

Caring people don't just happen. They are born out of the womb of God's eternal love for humanity, and become angels who walk among unnoticed. Elaine is one of those angels. Because they are embodied as one, Jason will reside in her heart and soul until the day they walk together throughout the eternal kingdom of God, never to be separated through time everlasting.. What happens inside the deep chasm of the mind and soul of those who are believers will forever belong to God.

Her deep faith and personal relationship with God prepared her to sustain the hope, strength, and bravery she needed. Was it only coincidence, that in the midst of her pain, she met so many strangers with unmistakable signs of something supernatural was taking place within the confines of this healing place.

She was Jason's mother, but she was also his hero. His love, kindness, and bravery, helped her to realize that there are times when the laws that govern life sometimes conclude without the assurance of divine intervention. She is among countless stoic mothers who live with shattered memories and visions of a life that once was, and although time doesn't always heal a broken heart, it provides us with strength slowly to move on, while healing their scars of pain and suffering

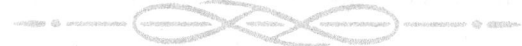

When Jason was born, I cried tears of Joy. When he died, I shed tears of sorrow and entered a into a nightmarish world that only those who have lost a child can understand; for it is not just the person you lose, but the many years of promise that will never be. Shareing my story is a step closer to healing, and I pray that anyone who has experienced such a tragic loss will find some small measure of comfort in the words I say. I feel your agony, and believe that nothing in this world truly ever belongs to any of us.

God bless you,
Elaine Coughlin

Author's Bio

Drake Gaetano is an author, poet, and humanitarian with an artistic soul. His writing career began as a blogger, capturing a wide audience in his pursuit of global peace. He is a prolific storyteller, an admitted small-town country boy who draws from his extensive background in the beauty industry as well as his personal life experiences to engage his readers.

Drake and his wife of 45 years live in a restored 1850s farmhouse on eight acres of land with Morgan horses, two golden doodles, and a cat. They are blessed with two grown children and one beloved grandson.

Borrowed Angel is Drake's third novel.

www.ingramcontent.com/pod-product-compliance
Lightning Source LLC
LaVergne TN
LVHW051925060526
838201LV00062B/4696